Common Murmurs, Arrhythmias and Myopathies of the Heart

A Collection of Cardiac Book Titles By Jim Lowrance

By: James M. Lowrance © 2012

TABLE OF CONTENTS/SECTIONS:

Common Murmurs, Arrhythmias and Myopathies of the Heart

INTRODUCTION:

This book of 17 chapters (approx. 19,650 words) is a compilation containing three of my previously published titles.

The section on common ectopic heartbeats (PVCs and PACs), is a subject that is also covered within a chapter of the section regarding heart problems associated with thyroid diseases as well but with added viewpoints.

It is important to note that according to thyroid disease medical sources, including the AACE (American Association of Clinical Endocrinologists), half of the American population with thyroid disease, remained undiagnosed and this number is in the tens-of-millions and tremendously higher when worldwide statistics are considered. This is why I have included the section regarding heart conditions that are thyroid disease related.

4

The information presented, can be of importance to anyone who is seeking to be heart-healthier and who is seeking to recognize signs and symptoms of the cardiac conditions that are discussed and treatments that are recommended/administered for them.

I have endeavored to provide a good general educational resource on these common conditions affecting cardiac function, with some being benign and others being potentially serious or even life-threatening. It is my sincere hope that readers find helpful information within the pages of this book.

-Jim Lowrance

SECTION ONE:

A Complete Look at Mitral Valve Prolapse Syndrome

The World's Most Common Heart Murmur

TABLE OF CONTENTS:

INTRODUCTION

Mitral Valve Prolapse is a heart murmur found commonly in the general public and can cause heart palpitations, orthostatic hypotension (dizziness upon standing), other symptoms of an imbalanced nervous system and anxiety/panic symptoms. Medical Research studies have found it to be even more common in thyroid disease patients, especially in those with autoimmune type thyroid disorders. It is also believed to be about 5 times more common in females than in males.

Many people with MVP do not experience symptoms while those who do are termed as having "MVP-Syndrome". The condition can also cause an imbalance in the "involuntary nervous system"(dysautonomia) and has been associated with Chronic Fatigue Syndrome in some patients who have it.

Interestingly a heart murmur was detected in me as a teen in the 1970s and they diagnosed it at a cardiologist's office as Wolf-Parkinson-White Syndrome.

This is a potentially serious type of heart murmur but over 20 years later at age 38 I had a new Cardiologist rule out my ever having WPWS. I had only an EKG/Stress Test conducted by the more recent cardiologist and Mitral Valve Prolapse is usually only detected by echocardiogram (ultrasound imaging), which I didn't request, nor was it recommended by the heart specialist.

I knew nothing about MVP at the time but after extensive search online, I realized that this is what I was experiencing for all of those years and that I still have symptoms-of, to this day. The nervous system related symptoms of the "syndrome" caused by MVP, in fact worsened in my case to some degree with the onset of autoimmune thyroid disease. I at times believe my CFS (Chronic Fatigue Syndrome) diagnosis, which was co morbid to my treated thyroid disorder also has MVPS as a major contributing factor.

CHAPTER ONE

How MVP-Syndrome May Manifest

The following two stories are fictitious examples, written by me – the author, to serve as examples of how one might discover that they are suffering from Mitral Valve Prolapse Syndrome.

Example Scenario One

"*I have the Mitral Valve Prolapse heart murmur. My doctor found it after I went to see him suffering with my heart fluttering and skipping. I had experienced irregular heartbeats for many years but the day it became severe for me was a day I returned home from a bicycle ride.*

I was riding on a trail with my daughter strapped in a booster seat on the back and I became unusually out of breath. When I stopped to rest I noticed my heart was beating at an incredible speed which scared the daylights out of me.

It's not unusual for me to get my heart rate to about 160 or 170 when I'm going max speed but on this day I was peddling only about mid speed and my heart was beating at least 200 BPM. Once I rested for a while it slowed to about 80 BPM but started skipping and fluttering about every third beat afterward, so my fear continued and I made an appointment to see my GP doctor. I was lucky that there was a cancellation by someone whose appointment I was able to be worked into.

My doctor questioned me about whether I smoked and I said no. He then asked if I drank a lot of caffeine or alcohol and to this I answered a big YES. I'm a notorious coffee addict and it is not unusual for me to drink 4 to 6 cups a day of strong Columbian dark roast. He listened to my heart and the flutters were obvious, so he sent me home with a pack containing 2 pills that I believe were called Atenolol that helped to reduce my elevated heart rate and it also stopped most of the fluttering beats. He wrote me an order to have a heart ultrasound done the next day and the Mitral Valve Prolapse was found clearly.

*He assured me that taking the low dose drug that
helped me and that he wrote me a refill
prescription for, would help my heart stay at a
regular rhythm. He said it was important not to
drink more than one cup of caffeinated coffee per
day and to eliminate it completely if possible or
switch to a decaffeinated brand and that I should
sleep regular and keep my stress level down. He
also recommended that I stay well hydrated by
drinking plenty of water. I continue to exercise
but do so, starting at a slow pace and I'm careful
not to exceed my tolerance level for physical
exertion. So far, these things have greatly helped
and I now have only rare symptoms from the
murmur. I hope my story helps others to have
hope with this condition."*

Example Scenario Two

"Back in my childhood I had a heart murmur but the doctor who found it said it didn't sound serious and that I would likely outgrow it. I always had palpitations and funny, fluttery heart beats in my chest but when I became hyperthyroid at age 41 from Grave's Disease the heart flutters starting getting severe and frightening because they were happening about every third or fourth beat of my heart.

I also began to experience serious anxiety symptoms and occasional panic attacks. My doctor ordered blood panels and found that I had Grave's Disease with a mildly overactive thyroid gland. I've been fortunate because mine was successfully controlled through anti-thyroid medication and so far I do not need my thyroid removed or killed off with radiation treatments.

I was also sent for a heart ultrasound and they found Mitral Valve Prolapse which was the cause of my heart murmur symptoms.

My hyperthyroid symptoms are much better but the heart skips are there about a third of the time and can become worse if I drink alcohol or too much caffeinated foods and beverages. I also get very dizzy and sometimes feel faint when I rise from sitting down and I get really short of breath and very tired when I exercise beyond short walks.

I'm on a beta-blocker blood pressure control drug which helps with a lot of this. I also take as-needed anti-anxiety medication when symptoms of anxiousness or panic becomes difficult for me to cope with. My doctor says I may never have to have my thyroid removed but that most people do end up having it done because the hyperthyroidism tends to return and becomes difficult to control with drugs alone. I hope in my case this doesn't happen but I will keep getting scheduled checkups so that any sign of more hyperthyroidism is hopefully stopped before reaching a point of my needing another procedure done."

The preceding two example scenarios are typical of those who first recognize the onset of Mitral Valve Prolapse Syndrome. For some of these people, they knew they had heart murmurs, many years in advance of experiencing any symptoms from it (usually recognized by doctors during their childhoods).

Some MVPS patients experience severe, ongoing symptoms that actually become disabling to them, to varying degrees. The two fictitious, example patients described above, would likely be in the area of MVPS symptom-manifestation that would fall somewhere between moderate and severe.

Regardless however, of how severe the symptoms of this common heart murmur may become, there are treatments and lifestyle changes that are very effective in controlling and in some cases alleviating MVPS symptoms. These will be discussed, in addition to further detail in regard to symptoms and diagnosis in the chapters that follow.

Keep in mind if you have dental work done, your Dentist may need to place you on antibiotics for a week or so before having procedures done, depending on whether or not you are experiencing mitral regurgitation and how severe it is (check with your doctor). This is because with some cases of MVP you may be at higher risk for infection and inflammation developing in and around your heart (carditis), after undergoing dental work. This is only a risk if a significant degree of blood-seepage from it is occurring, meaning the mitral valve is regurgitating/leaking significant amounts of blood, due to inadequate sealing of it during heart contractions.

CHAPTER TWO

Basics about Mitral Valve Prolapse Syndrome

MVP itself, is a common condition of the heart that can cause concerning symptoms in some patients who experience it, at which point, it is called "Mitral Valve Prolapse Syndrome" as previously mentioned. Other patients with the same heart condition do not have symptoms from it and in this case, it is simply referred to as "Mitral Valve Prolapse" (drop the "Syndrome" off the end of the term). Abbreviated, the terms are "MVP" and "MVPS".

Both symptomatic and asymptomatic cases of MVP are usually benign conditions in the vast majority of cases, meaning they do not progress to harmful or life-threatening conditions for most patients, although these risks do increase in the elderly.

In this chapter, I want to again address MVPS, the category of the heart murmur that causes symptoms.

It is also called a "click murmur" due to a clicking sound that can sometimes be heard coming from the heart, by use of a stethoscope by a medical professional, who monitors each beat. The clicking-sound according to medical sources, is caused by the "Mitral Valve Leaflets" becoming somewhat stretched out, so that they are slightly loose or they develop scar tissue on them and become slightly thickened and both of these manifestations can cause them to have a slight vibration-effect, as the heartbeats. This may also cause mild, moderate or severe "regurgitation" (blood seepage from the valve) that is picked up as a more prominent clicking sound (murmur) or that is accompanied by a "swishing" type sound, with a stethoscope.

Other patients may not have a clicking sound that is as easily heard through a stethoscope but if symptoms being experienced, point to MVP, a more sensitive test may be ordered for detection of the murmur, called an "Echocardiogram".

This test uses the same principle as a Sonogram that women who are pregnant have administered, to monitor the progress of their baby's development within the womb. Sound waves are sent into the area to be observed and they are transmitted as an image onto a screen, so that even the tiniest movement in the heart can be seen. This is how patients with more difficult to detect MVP, can be diagnosed or have the condition ruled out as a cause of their symptoms.

Severe cases of MVP may cause a more severe form of "regurgitation", meaning the blood-leakage from the valves is more significant, with heartbeats. Heart valves of course are supposed to be self-contained, so that blood flows through them without leakage but with MVP-Regurgitation, blood does escape from the valve and this form of the murmur will sometimes require surgery to be corrected, However, it is a rare form of MVP, with elderly patients being at higher risk for its development, as previously mentioned.

Following are some of the symptoms that may occur with MVP, placing the murmur into the "syndrome" category (MVP-S).

• a racing heart (tachycardia)
• heart skips and flutters (PVCs and PACs)
• fatigue
• dizziness
• shortness of breath
• anxiety symptoms, including panic attacks
• orthostatic hypotension (dizzy upon standing from a seated or lying down position)
• sensitivities to chemicals (i.e. caffeine, alcohol, tobacco, chocolate and refined sugar)

The chemical sensitivities I list above are triggers that can cause worsening of symptoms in some patients with MVPS. The Orthostatic Hypotension, also called "Orthostatic Intolerance", is also classified as a form of "Dysautonomia", meaning a slight deregulation of the "Involuntary Nervous System" (INS) is occurring.

Some medical researchers believe that the dysautonomia found in some MVP patients, is what actually causes the syndrome aspect (MVP-S) due to the Involuntary Nervous System playing a major role in regulating heart rate and blood pressure. When it becomes deregulated due to MVP, this is what causes symptoms, resulting in the syndrome, according to these sources. The heart murmur itself may be mild and still result in an array of symptoms and so how severe they are, does not necessarily indicate a severe case of MVP. The reverse scenario may also be true in some patients and a severe case of MVP may cause very few symptoms but this is less common than are mild cases that cause significant symptoms.

In regard to anxiety symptoms found in MVPS, it has been long known that MVP is notorious for causing chronic anxiety and panic attacks and many patients are actually diagnosed with Anxiety Disorders, due to this underlying medical condition.

If patients can find control of the symptoms of MVPS through proper treatment and coping methods, the anxiety symptoms will also be alleviated to a large degree, if not completely resolved. More in regard to anxiety symptoms associated with MVP will be specifically addressed within the chapters that follow.

CHAPTER THREE

More about MVP Symptoms

Palpitations - If you notice that you have episodes of skipped heartbeats, heart flutters and flip-flops or rapid heartbeats (tachycardia), this can indicate that you have MVPS. The "skipping beats" aspect, is actually caused by "extra heartbeats" but that is felt as a pause by the one experiencing them. These come under the categories of "Premature Ventricular Contractions" (extra beats originating from the heart's lower chambers) and "Premature Atrial Contractions" (originating from the heart's upper chambers) and both types are usually benign (harmless) in the vast majority of cases.

The irregular heartbeats caused by MVPS are due to slight abnormalities in the mitral valve leaflets, or the supporting valve chords, or both. These structures allow the leaflet(s) to prolapse (or buckle) back into the left atrium during the heart's contraction-ventricular systole.

While medical research has not concluded definitively what causes the mitral valve to prolapse abnormally in some people, they theorize that it is due to these valve leaflets becoming either thickened or stretched out over time and this causes them to vibrate or quiver slightly as previously mentioned, causing the "click murmur".

Anxiety - If you are experiencing panic attacks, frequent episodes of free-floating anxiety (high, prolonged levels) or depression symptoms, with no apparent cause for them, this may indicate that you have MVPS, especially if one or more of the other symptoms as listed previously are also present.

Anxiety is one of the more frightening symptoms of MVPS because panic attacks especially, are the more common type of anxiety that people with this disorder experience. Medical research is not clear as to how anxiety symptoms are caused by MVPS, but some sources state that it could be due to slightly abnormal electrical impulses in the heart, caused by the abnormal prolapsing of the mitral valve leaflets.

This triggers the "fight or flight response" more frequently or at inappropriate and unexpected times (adrenaline rush designed to help us fight or to flee from danger when the need arises).

While anxiety is listed more commonly for MVPS, depression is also experienced frequently in patients with the click murmur. Patients may find that they frequently experience both of these emotions simultaneously or they may find that these alternate, so that they are experiencing anxiety at some times and depression at other times.

Hypotension - Dizziness in general and dizziness upon standing from a sitting or lying down position (supine) can mean that you are experiencing spells of low blood pressure, low blood volume (hypovolemia) or possibly an ongoing problem with inadequate blood pressure regulation (the needed increases and decreases with physical activities), which can indicate that you have MVPS.

The term for getting dizzy upon first rising, after sitting or lying down is "orthostatic hypotension" and is a form of "dysautonomia," which is a medical term for an irregular response by the involuntary nervous system. This system of the body, also referred to as the "autonomic nervous system" automatically regulates our involuntary bodily functions, such as heart rate, respiration and blood pressure changes with physical activities. It also regulates our breathing (especially during sleep) and keeps all of our bodily organs and glands functioning correctly (i.e. the liver, kidneys, brain and endocrine system).

Certain diseases and disorders, including MVPS, can cause this system of our body to operate abnormally, which can result in blood pressure not rising enough upon standing (hypotension) to supply adequate blood circulation to the heart and brain. While this irregular response usually only lasts a few seconds, it can also make a person with MVPS feel faint, dizzy and pressure-type sensations in the head and neck.

This dysautonomia aspect may also be the cause of the anxiety symptoms addressed in the previous subheading, according to some medical sources (More on this condition in CHAPTER FOUR).

Breathlessness - If you become short of breath more easily and have less tolerance for exercise and physical exertion, this may indicate that you have MVPS. Of course this can also be a sign of pulmonary conditions (lung disease) or a number of other health disorders, so as with all other symptoms being discussed, it must have professional medical evaluation given to it.

People with MVPS will find that they become fatigued more easily from exercise and physical exertion and that they become short of breath more easily as well. Tolerance for exercise can become noticeably lowered in people with MVPS when they are experiencing the onset of symptoms they have not previously experienced with physical exertion.

This syndrome can have an onset (symptom flares) at any age according to medical sources, however symptoms are more common in women and more commonly found in ages beginning in the mid-teens and older. Some MVPS patients may find that everyday activities fatigue them more easily and more often than before experiencing the onset of the syndrome.

Chemical Sensitivities - If you have become sensitive to caffeine, chocolate, alcohol, excess sugar and other stimulants, this may indicate you have MVPS. By "sensitivity", I am referring to negative reactions from these substances.

People who are experiencing MVPS find that they have unpleasant aftereffects from foods and drinks containing stimulant-type chemicals. Tobacco-use can also cause symptom flares, due to nicotine and other chemicals it contains. These sensitive people will find that overindulgence of these chemicals or that even small to moderate amounts of any type stimulant can cause them symptom-reactions.

Even an extra cup of coffee or a chocolate bar can cause their heart to skip beats or flutter and can also trigger anxiety attacks, depression and fatigue more easily. We could also add "stress" to this category because stress is stimulating and a necessary mechanism in our daily lives however, stress levels that are excessive or prolonged can cause the same symptom flares in MVPS patients that other stimulants can.

While a patient will notice the symptoms previously listed, before they suspect that MVPS could be the cause, these are the observations that should prompt a visit to a licensed physician. Once a patient has described their symptoms to their doctor in-detail, he can perform a physical, including listening very closely to the patient's heart.

He may be able to detect a heart murmur by stethoscope but in many cases, MVP cannot be detected unless the patient is sent (referred) to a cardiologist/heart specialist for an echocardiogram.

By use of the very sensitive sound waves transmitted onto a screen via this test, the function of the heart can be monitored very clearly. If a patient has Mitral Valve Prolapse, the condition will usually be more definitively detected and diagnosed using this imaging test.

CHAPTER FOUR

More about Orthostatic Hypotension

Orthostatic Hypotension (OH) is a common condition that causes the one experiencing it to feel dizzy and/or faint when first standing-up. If this effect lasts for longer periods of time or worsens, the longer a person stands, it may then be referred to as "Orthostatic Intolerance". Most cases of this condition are mild and not harmful or difficult to treat. In most cases, any actual danger the condition poses is the risk of experiencing injury from a fall, due to becoming dizzy or faint when it occurs.

The condition is also experienced commonly by thyroid patients, especially those with Grave's disease but it can also occur with hypothyroid states when blood pressure and heart rate become inadequate. People with blood glucose problems, such as hypoglycemia (sudden drops in blood sugar levels), people who are fully diabetic and those who become dehydrated or anemic, can also experience symptoms of OH.

It can become a feature of other dysautonomic conditions as well, including Mitral Valve Prolapse Syndrome and Postural Orthostatic Tachycardia Syndrome (POTS).

Orthostatic Hypotension (OH) by itself is also a form of dysautonomia. When a person experiences a problem with their involuntary nervous system (INS), the result can be one of a number of conditions that fall under the dysautonomia category, including OH. This means that involuntary bodily functions such as heart beat, breathing and blood pressure regulation, become imbalanced due to not being sufficiently regulated by the INS. As a result the condition may cause a variety of symptoms.

The different variations of Orthostatic Hypotension are defined when one experiences sudden drops in blood pressure when first standing or a continued worsening of low blood pressure during periods of standing. Other medical names for the condition include "Postural Hypotension" and "Neurally Mediated Hypotension".

As previously mentioned, most people with this condition experience a sudden but temporary drops in blood pressure when first standing-up from lying down (supine) or from a seated position. The INS is supposed to maintain blood pressure with changes in body positions and should actually cause a temporary, mild rise in blood pressure when standing up, in order to move blood from the lower extremities, to the upper part of the body.

There are a number of other symptoms that can occur with OH, in addition to those already mentioned. In most cases, the drops in blood pressure after standing from supine positions usually lasts a few seconds, with symptoms occurring, only as long as it takes for the blood pressure to normalize but rarely, the problem can be prolonged and ongoing (chronic).

If this bodily response is mildly, moderately or severely hindered by an imbalance in the INS, the symptoms experienced may also include the following. ---

---

- dizziness
- headache
- blurred vision
- nausea
- increased heart rate (tachycardia)
- possible fainting (syncope)

Some people with OH also report experiencing spells of fatigue from this condition, especially after repeated episodes of OH when their activities require a great deal of postural changes throughout the day.

While dysautonomia from MVPS is a common cause for OH, other things that can contribute-to or serve as a cause for an abnormal INS, include other types of heart conditions (including other less commonly experienced murmurs and overt heart failure), certain medications, adrenal insufficiency, neurological diseases and low sodium (salt) in the body. Other types of chronic diseases and illnesses that require prolonged bed rest can also be a cause of OH and dysautonomia.

Treatment for OH depends on its severity. Most people have mild cases and their doctors will prescribe a healthy diet, exercise and adequate rest and sleep to help with the condition. In more severe cases, medications may be prescribed to help regulate the abnormal fluctuations in blood pressure. An increase in sodium (salt) intake may be also suggested by a doctor if hypertension is not also present. An increase in fluid intake might also be suggested, to help keep blood volume at adequate levels in the body, if chronic heart failure is not also present.

Medications that might be administered to an OH patient might include blood pressure regulating drugs such as beta blockers, mineral corticosteroids (a type of cortisol steroid) and/or drugs that stimulate the nervous system. Other patients may be prescribed drugs such as amphetamines or ephedrine, which help to increase adrenaline levels in the body. The type of treatment is based upon how severely the symptoms of OH are affecting the patient.

Cases that are mild to moderate can usually be treated with the diet modifications and lifestyle changes previously mentioned.

If you experience symptoms of OH, it is important to make an office visit with to a qualified medical doctor to determine the cause and to receive treatment that is best suited for your case.

CHAPTER FIVE

More about Treatment for Mitral Valve Prolapse

There are treatments and lifestyle changes for MVPS that can reduce or eliminate its symptoms significantly in most cases. I addressed the symptoms of this disorder in the previous chapters as well but I will again briefly list those most frequently experienced in a bit more detail. To repeat, the main symptoms of the syndrome can include; rapid heart rate, heart skips and flip-flops, fatigue, dizziness upon standing, anxiety, depression and chemical sensitivities.

What are the more common treatments prescribed for Mitral Valve Prolapse when is causes symptoms? According to statistics this common condition affecting as much as 20% of the U.S. population,usually requires no medical treatment because most patients do not experience significant symptoms (MVP-Syndrome).

For the majority of those who do experience symptoms, they do not require actual pharmaceutical treatments but when a Doctor does prescribe a drug for highly symptomatic patients, it will often be a "Beta-Blocker" because the drug can help to control a number of symptoms that may be present. This drug counteracts the stimulatory effects of adrenaline (epinephrine). In other words, it partially blocks some of the effects of the hormone adrenaline, thereby controlling the rapid heart rate, wide blood pressure fluctuations and the related anxiety symptoms.

More severe cases of MVPS, which are rare, sometimes require surgical procedures to repair defective valves but for the majority of patients, symptoms are controlled through diet, exercise and natural or prescribed supplements.

The diet aspect would be to avoid stimulants in the diet as listed previously that can act as triggers for MVPS symptoms and flares.

A healthy diet should include lots of fruits, vegetables, nuts and grains (complex carbohydrates) which are always a good idea, as opposed to junk foods (simple carbohydrates) that can only serve to quickly stimulate the body, followed by crashes in energy levels. Also a good multi-vitamin helps the body's systems operate at a more optimal level, without the wide stimulating effects.

MVP patients should also take a "magnesium" supplement – a mineral that helps keep heart function healthy but they may first need to have their magnesium blood level checked (or other method of mineral analysis) to see how much they need to be taking and to only take the amount recommended by their doctor. Taking the RDA (recommended Daily Allowance) of magnesium is usually safe for anyone but with MVPS, a doctor may prescribe higher supplementation amounts.

Exercise is also greatly helpful in regulating the "Involuntary Nervous System" (highly involved in heart function), blood-pressure and anxiety symptoms. It can also help reduce stress levels that often contribute to symptoms associated with MVPS and dysautonomia. Exercise can be of more benefit than any other single factor of treatment in many cases but a patient must pace their self and only exercise at their tolerance-level, afterward, slowly increasing the level as they are able to do so. Walking is a great way to begin an exercise program and even if you only increase the distance and/or briskness of your walk, slowly over time, the benefits can be tremendous.

CHAPTER SIX

Strong Association of Thyroid Disease to MVP

Some medical research articles state that MVP is a common finding in thyroid disease patients, which could mean that thyroid disease may be one of several possible triggers for this syndrome or it may aggravate the condition in people who already had MVP, prior to the onset of their thyroid diseases. I have done extensive search and research on this connection and have found no less than five highly reputable research groups reporting on this association. What does this mean for thyroid patients?

The medical reports themselves state that this fact demonstrates the importance for thyroid patients in being tested for this heart murmur. Some of the research states the possibility that MVP also has an autoimmune component to it or that it may be an autoimmune disease itself. Some of the symptoms related to this heart murmur, are a result of "dysautonomia", as previously mentioned.

It is possible that people who already have MVP but who also experience the onset of an autoimmune thyroid disease (Graves' disease or Hashimoto's thyroiditis), can see the MVP/MVPS worsen in symptom manifestations. It is also possible that thyroid autoimmunity itself, serves as a trigger for causing MVPS.

These strong possibilities must be considered because medical research conclusions have shown the condition to be very common in thyroid patients, as opposed to control groups (non thyroid disease participants).

Professor Bell, director of the endocrine clinic at the University Of Alabama School Of Medicine in Birmingham, AL for example; has reported finding MVP present in 41% of patients with Hashimoto's thyroiditis and in 41% of Graves ' disease patients who were studied. (Source: WebMD)

Professor M.E. Evangelopoulou and colleagues from Alexandra Hospital at Athens University School of Medicine reported an average of 1 in 4 patients with Graves' and Hashimoto's, as having co morbid (associated) MVP.

None of the healthy people in the control group without thyroid disease were found to have MVP. (Study Title: Heart Valve Defect Common in Patients with Thyroid Disease)

The American Journal of Psychiatry published a study in 1987 that states there is strongly confirmed association between panic attacks, mitral valve prolapse, and autoimmune thyroid disorders. (Study Title: Mitral Valve prolapse and thyroid abnormalities in patients with panic attacks)

Several studies are also published on the U.S. National Institutes of Health-National Library of Medicine medical research website (PubMed).

One of the studies states that *"the prevalence of mitral valveprolapse is significantly increased in patients with autoimmune disorders of the thyroid gland, when compared to normals and nonautoimmune conditions"* (Study Title: Prevalence of mitral valve prolapse in chronic lymphocytic thyroiditis and nongoitrous hypothyroidism.)

Another important aspect to this subject is the fact that thyroid patients, who have MVP/MVPS, may in-fact confuse the symptoms of the heart murmur with unresolved thyroid disease symptoms or with under-treated hypothyroidism. Some medical sources out there also state that people with MVPS may sometimes be diagnosed as having Chronic Fatigue Syndrome (CFS). Another connection regarding CFS is the fact that people suffering the condition often have dysautonomia which is also a common finding in MVPS.

I personally see in this subject of MVP being strongly associated with autoimmune thyroid disease, the importance in recognizing how commonly co morbid some conditions are.

It also points to the importance in considering these connections when thyroid patients are not experiencing the expected symptom relief from their treatments. Doctors should recognize the need in testing for MVPS in these patients whose unresolved symptoms match those for this common heart murmur.

CHAPTER SEVEN

Book Review: MVPS-Dysautonomia Survival Guide

(NOTE: I originally wrote this book review for the BellaOnline Thyroid health site.)

The full title of the book is *"The Mitral Valve Prolapse Syndrome/Dysautonomia Survival Guide"* and this is my review for this highly-informative book. I highly recommended it to my readers at BellaOnline Thyroid Health. When corresponding with the authors, I made mention that I hear from many thyroid patients who have Mitral Valve Prolapse and the related syndrome and they acknowledged hearing from many thyroid patients with the condition as well. I'm grateful for the free copy of the book they sent me for reviewing.

I finished reading this incredible book, the month of February, 2009 and was actually disappointed when I came to the end of it because it was such an interesting read!

James and Cheryl Durante have authored this book, along with John G. Furiasse, MD, a director of a medical center in Illinois that brilliantly covers all of the important aspects of a condition called "Mitral Valve Prolapse Syndrome". This common heart murmur that is not widely recognized by the medical community as being significant but that is gaining recognition with each passing year, can seriously affect those who have the syndrome it may cause.

The authors give a detailed but easy-to-understand description of Mitral Valve Prolapse (MVP) itself with professional line-art drawings included in the book, to show the reader how the mitral valves in the heart and the mitral leaflets extending from them are affected by this condition. They also help the reader to understand the difference between MVP, which is the condition apart from the symptoms it causes and Mitral Valve Prolapse Syndrome (MVPS) -- the name used for the condition when it does cause symptoms.

The book leads the reader through a description of both the physical and psychological symptoms caused by MVPS and how these can seriously affect the quality of life in those who experience them.

The subject of "dysautonomia", a co-occurring imbalance in the function of the involuntary nervous system is addressed in detail as well in this book, which is believed to be a major cause of the symptom aspects of MVP-Syndrome. The physical symptoms that result from MVPS-Dysautonomia are thoroughly detailed, including its affects in causing imbalance in blood pressure regulation and in causing imbalances in both the "sympathetic" and "parasympathetic" systems of the nervous system. These systems are also what control the amount of adrenal hormone that is produced in the body and how often it is released in triggering the "fight or flight response" (anxiety mechanism) and how these involuntary systems also calm the body down after an alarm phase.

The authors point out that this imbalance aspect of MVPS-Dysautonomia is believed to be responsible for the anxiety problems experienced by those with the syndrome, resulting in panic attacks and other conditions of disordered anxiety.

Other problems may result as well, including ongoing and severe (chronic) fatigue, dizziness and exercise intolerance, which when all combined, can seriously affect the quality of life for those who suffer MVPS-Dysautonomia.

We then come to the part of the book that helps MVPS patients learn to cope-with and or even overcome the symptoms of this condition, thereby restoring a higher quality of life to them. A number of patient testimonials about symptom-struggles they have experienced from MVPS-Dysautonomia are included, as well as testimonials of recovery from these symptoms and ongoing positive improvement with proper treatment.

The authors detail medication-options for treating both the physical and emotional symptoms of MVPS-Dysautonomia but also describe available therapies, such as Cognitive Behavioral Therapy and Exposure Therapy to help with anxiety disorder and phobia struggles, as well as deep breathing and relaxation techniques. Also discussed in the book are methods for helping those who need help in regaining self-confidence and self-esteem that can also be seriously affected by MVPS-Dysautonomia.

I, the author of this review, have experienced the symptoms of MVPS-Dysautonomia since my teen years and possibly earlier and I related a great deal to the symptom descriptions contained in this book. I also know that both James and Cheryl Durante authored this book from the perspective of having experienced this condition as well which gives the reader a perspective of MVPS-Dysautonomia they can better relate to.

The book is available through major book sellers.

CHAPTER EIGHT

MVP a Medical cause of Anxiety Symptoms

This common condition I have described in the preceding chapters, that often causes a "click murmur" in the heart has been studied by medical groups and found to be a common cause of anxiety symptoms and panic attacks. Though statistics vary in regard to the number of Americans that have this disorder, one of the more commonly published statistics states that up to 1 in 5 Americans have varying degrees of Mitral Valve Prolapse.

While there have yet to be definitive reasons found for why this usually benign heart irregularity causes anxiety symptoms, there are several theories considered. The most accepted theory is that small, irregular changes in electrical impulses that take place in the heart that are regulated by the involuntary nervous system cause episodes of too much release of adrenaline from the adrenal glands.

The heart has many nerve impulses triggered within it that regulate the speed of heart function by interacting with the adrenal glands. With MVP, it is believed that these nerve impulses become irregular so that false signals indicating the need for increased heart rate reach the adrenal glands, causing excessive release of hormone (adrenaline surges).

Anxiety symptoms may include the following.

• apprehension
• worry
• feelings of fear
• rapid heart beat
• hyperventilation
• excessive sweating
• blushing
• trembling
• increased blood pressure
• muscle tension
• an urge to escape

Normally adrenaline is released to change the pace of the heart's beating to compensate for increased physical activity (sympathetic response) or when there is a change in body-posture, such as standing from a seated position (postural blood pressure changes).

With Mitral Valve Prolapse the irregular nerve impulses to the heart may trigger these adrenaline surges a bit more erratically, causing increased anxiety symptoms.

If you suspect that MVPS could be the cause of anxiety symptoms you are experiencing, the symptoms I've discussed can be observations that should prompt a visit to a medical physician.

Once a patient suspecting MVP can describe their symptoms to their doctor, he can perform a physical, including listening closely to the patient's heart and recommending specialized cardiac testing as needed.

A regular doctor (MD or GP) may detect MVP by stethoscope but in many cases, it cannot be detected unless the patient is sent to a cardiologist (heart specialist) for definitive tests. If a patient has Mitral Valve Prolapse, the condition will most likely be detected and definitively diagnosed using echo-imaging.

CHAPTER NINE

Coping with MVP-caused Panic Attacks and Severe Anxiety Episodes

A panic attack is a climax of anxiety symptoms that causes them to be experienced suddenly and forcefully. People, who experience frequent panic attacks, have a condition referred to as "Panic Disorder". The following four steps, listed under subheadings below, which are often used in different variations of "Cognitive Behavioral Therapy" (CBT) can help those who suffer panic attacks, to calm their selves when experiencing them.

Remind yourself during a panic attack, that you will not drop dead or lose your sanity.

While panic attacks are the most unpleasant type of anxiety that can be experienced, reputable mental health sources state that they do not lead to loss of sanity, strokes or heart attacks, in otherwise healthy people.

Anxiety is a normal mechanism, designed to give the body increased strength to escape danger or to fight an enemy should situations arise requiring the need to do so. It is also designed to help us accomplish urgent or important duties that life might present to us. Panic attacks are an example of this important mechanism, occurring "out of context" meaning they are triggered at times when there is no actual need for the "fight or flight" response to occur.

While this improper timing makes panic attacks extremely unpleasant, they are still a normal response the body is designed to experience without causing injury to the mind or body. The real damage chronic anxiety conditions result-in is restricting some of the freedom and enjoyments of life rather than actually causing mental or physical damage. Reminding yourself of these simple facts, can help diminish the effects of a panic attack and lend toward calming yourself down during one.

Focus on the task you are involved in rather than focusing on the panic attack symptoms.

While this step is certainly easier-said-than-done, with practice, you can learn to divert your attention away from the unpleasant anxiety symptoms/sensations and direct your focus more toward accomplishing an immediate goal at hand. The triggers that cause panic attacks can be simple things such as waiting in line to be checked out at a grocery store or walking to the front isle of a theater to be seated.

Other times things that cause panic attacks are of more importance and significance, such as standing before an audience to make an important speech or rescuing someone from a burning home. Regardless of the tasks needing performed, you can practice focusing more on accomplishing them than on the panic symptoms they may be triggering. This will channel your attention toward your energy in performing these tasks, rather than upon surviving the anxiety symptoms that are attempting to challenge you.

If you feel panic symptoms arising while being checked out at the grocery line, you might consider focusing intently on the magazines or other items near the checkout stand. When your groceries are being checked out, you might consider mentally calculating the total cost of your groceries to see how close you come to the final tally. If it helps to join in with the clerk in bagging the groceries, you might consider this as a diversion from focusing on anxiety symptoms. Any method that helps you divert your attention and energy into a task rather than focusing on the anxiety is acceptable and you can also make a game out of it, so that you look forward to the gains you will make over time and actually begin to enjoy accomplishing these goals.

Realize that you are not alone in experiencing panic attacks and that they are not a sign of weakness.

Panic attacks are experienced by an estimated 6 million Americans or about 1 out of every 75 people.

Mental health professionals who study anxiety disorders, including panic attacks, have found that people who suffer chronic anxiety, are many times the more creative and passionate people in our society. Famous sports figures including pro football players Earl Campbell and Ricky Williams have suffered panic attacks, as well as famous celebrities including Howie Mandel and Oprah Winfrey. This places people who suffer panic attacks and panic disorder in good company with some of our nation's most ambitious people. By reminding yourself that greatly-admired and creative people suffer chronic anxiety conditions, you can also view yourself as among the most creative and passionate people of our society.

Channel your anxiety into a positive and creative process.

Many anxiety sufferers have found that when they feel on-edge or as if they are on the verge of experiencing a panic attack, they are also at their most creative and passionate level.

By taking that anxiety energy and channeling it into positive actions, you can redirect it away from negative experiences. Rather than running from the anxiety symptoms or attempting to escape from them when they occur, try channeling that energy into creating something you enjoy.

If you enjoy sculpting, writing or painting, allow the anxiety to trigger your creative juices into flowing by concentrating that energy into those creative arts. If you enjoy sports, such as soccer, tennis or martial arts, channel that anxiety energy into improving upon your skills and techniques in these areas.

If you are involved in something or in a location where this is not possible to actually practice these past-times when anxiety symptoms occur, you might attempt to mentally play the sport in your mind or carry a small notepad for jotting-down notes on how you can improve in the sport when you are able to play again.

While the following final-suggestion for this step might seem unusual, I will mention that there is a UK website that recently reported that a PhD Stress Management Expert in the U.S. found that anxiety and stress relief can be experienced using romantic and sexual fantasy as an anxiety diversion technique.

In his research, he found that people who conjure torrid fantasies involving romantic and sexual scenarios have found that it helps them to divert negative anxiety responses into passionate imagination, with positive results. I would also add the suggestion that you use your spouse and life partner as the object of your fantasies, which will improve both your anxiety symptoms and your love life at the same time.

These are examples of things that can help to diminish the effects of anxiety symptoms and that can also help those who suffer panic attacks, to redirect their anxiety into a positive rather than into a negative direction and outcome.

Treatment for anxiety and other symptoms of MVP may also include beta-blocker medications that help control the effects of adrenaline in the body as mentioned previously and/or anti-anxiety and antidepressant medications.

Types of anti-anxiety medications (benzodiazepines) include the following:
• alprazolam (Xanax®)
• clonazepam (Klonipin®)
• lorazepam (Ativan®)
• diazepam (Valium®)

• buspirone (Buspar®) (this one is a azaspirodecanedione class drug)

Types of anti-depressants (selective serotonin reuptake inhibitors) that also work as anti-anxiety medications include the following:
• paroxetine (Paxil®)
• venlafexine (Effexor®)
• fluoxetine (Prozac®)
• setraline (Zoloft®)
• fluvoxamine (Luvox ®)

The lifestyle and diet changes discussed in previous chapters can also significantly contribute to relief of anxiety symptoms and it is my sincere hope that the preceding information proves to be helpful to the readers of it.

(END - SECTION ONE)

SECTION TWO:

Are Common Heart Skip Palpitations Dangerous?

Premature Ventricular and Atrial Contractions (PVCs and PACs)

TABLE OF CONTENTS:

INTRODUCTION:

Skipped heartbeats occur in most, if not 100% of the general population, at some point during their lives. Some medical sources state that about half of us experience them on a relatively frequent basis. For some people however, these heart palpitations called "Premature Ventricular Contractions" and "Premature Atrial Contractions" (PVCs and PACs), occur at a frequency or forcefulness, that can be concerning to them and that can result in chronic anxiety and/or panic attacks. In most cases these palpitations are benign but the unpleasant feeling they may cause can at times override any reassurance one might receive by a doctor, that their heart is otherwise healthy and normal.

It would seem that some individuals are more aware of their skipped heartbeats than are others, which in-reality are extra heartbeats (extra systole: ectopic heartbeats) that cause the sensation of missed ones. Many people with PVCs and/or PACs, are finely tuned-in to the symptoms these may cause.

Once anxiety over them is added, they can occur with more force and frequency (in most cases anxiety and stress precedes and triggers them). While this still does not make them dangerous, according to many reputable heart specialists, the fear and anticipation of them can degrade a person's quality of life. It in-essence becomes an anxiety disorder in itself or is added to an existing one, causing a worsening of symptoms.

It is my intention, through the chapters of this book, to inform readers who experience these common but most-often benign palpitations, with facts, that can help them to better-cope with the concerning symptoms they may experience with these strange heartbeats.

CHAPTER ONE

Understanding Premature Ventricular and Atrial Contractions

Just Exactly What are these Heart Skip Palpitations?

Premature Ventricular Contractions (PVCs - originating from the lower heart valves) and Premature Atrial Contractions (PACs - originating from the upper heart valves) are mild and usually benign cardiac events, that can cause some degree of symptoms but that are usually not life restricting, other than the possible mental stress and anxiety that can accompany them.

While people who experience these disrhythmias are usually at no risk for any type of negative consequence from experiencing them, many will find it very hard not to be concerned about them, even after reassurance by their medical doctors, who inform them that the palpitations (unusual sensations from the heart), are harmless.

66

I cannot fault those individuals who do experience anxiety resulting from PVCs and/or PACS because I personally began to experience these skipping heartbeats, in my teen years and because of the very unusual feeling they produced, which can be described as a pause in heartbeats, followed by a thump-sensation in the chest. Mine have continued to occur intermittently and I am now one birthday away from being 50 years old at the time of this writing. So far, I have seen no ill effect from them, other than the panic and anxiety symptoms I have experienced with them on occasion. Now, when I begin to see them manifest, I can usually ignore them, since gaining the knowledge that they are harmless in the vast majority of cases, although I will admit that when they occur with frequency or in multiples, I can still find myself feeling anxious.

I actually made an office visit with a cardiologist in the year 2001, after experiencing a long period of frequent PVCs/PACs and my results from a stress electrocardiogram, showed no abnormalities in my heart rhythm or any suspected blockage in any of my heart vessels or valves.

Another reason I scheduled the visit with a heart specialist, was due to my being diagnosed with a heart murmur, in my teens. A medical doctor, who was treating me at the time for a condition unrelated to my heart, heard the murmur during my visit with him, at about age 15. He informed my parents and recommended that we schedule an appointment with a cardiologist. Upon being examined and having heart testing conducted, including an EKG, a heart exray and cardiac ultrasound (echocardiogram), the cardiologist concluded that I was experiencing "Wolff-Parkinson-White Syndrome" (WPWS); a potentially serious heart murmur. He explained to both my parents and me, that this meant that I basically had an extra electrical pathway in my heart, that was causing a faster rhythm or what is also referred to as "tachycardia". He also informed us that he felt the murmur was of a mild variety in the category of the heart murmur.

The cardiologist I saw in 2001, stated that the previous diagnosis was incorrect because the murmur was not found during the more recent testing and that the previous heart specialist was mistaken.

He informed me that he specializes in cases of WPWS and that he had published studies he was involved with, in researching the murmur and that if I actually had the condition, it would still be present and unchanged without surgical correction of it. While I was relieved to receive the all-clear more than 20 years later, I now realize that the diagnosis I was given in my teens, caused me to become more "heartbeat conscious". My fear of the heart murmur, was causing me to monitor my cardiac activity much closer and I found myself taking my pulse frequently and paying close attention to the speed of my heart rhythm.

I had actually begun to experience infrequent episodes of panic sensations even previous to my knowledge of having the heart murmur, which I apparently outgrew or that was misdiagnosed. I also began to have ongoing problems with free-floating anxiety as well (generalized feelings of anxiousness), which became chronic as years passed and that eventually fit the definition of "generalized Anxiety Disorder", by the time I reached 19 years of age.

This is also the approximate time I began experiencing the heart-skip palpitations, which genuinely caused me to fear what was occurring within my heart. I attributed these to the heart murmur and I believed this to be the case for nearly two decades before receiving the counter-diagnoses at age 38. My episodes of the skipping heartbeats, would occur following long episodes of stress or anxiety or after I had consumed too many stimulants in my diet (i.e. caffeine, alcohol or refined sugars). I noticed that I would experience them for days, weeks or even for months at a time, with periods of relief from them in-between, that were months or even years in duration. I now believe that these symptoms I was experiencing, including the tachycardia as a teen, were actually caused by a condition known as "Mitral Valve Prolapse" (MVP), which is a common murmur found in the general population and that can become a "syndrome" (MVPS), when symptoms are caused by it.

In addition to heart skip palpitations and heart rhythm changes, MVP-Syndrome, can result in symptoms of dizziness, sensitivities to stimulants, fatigue, blood pressure changes (usually low -- hypotension) and shortness of breath.

Common Murmurs, Arrhythmias and Myopathies of the Heart

I also believe MVP to be the heart murmur that was originally detected in me, due to both of my parents having been diagnosed with it in their 70s and my daughter being diagnosed with a benign heart murmur in her pre-teens (it is highly hereditary). MVP itself, which is also referred to as a "click murmur" (describing the sound it sometimes produces when monitored by stethoscope), is also a usually-benign condition but that is notorious for causing heart skip palpitations (more on MVP/MVPS later).

I feel that my previous diagnoses of WPWS, began a vicious cycle of increased anxiety for me, which led to my experiences with PVCs/PACs. The sensation of a pause in the heartbeat caused by these disrhythmias is actually caused by "extra heartbeats", also referred to as "ectopic" and "extrasystole" heartbeats. These can be fairly rare in occurrence for many people or they may occur with relative frequency however, even the latter is not usually of concern in the vast majority of cases. Some individuals may also experience them, with every other heartbeat (bigeminy) or every third heartbeat (trigeminy) or every fourth heartbeat (quadrigeminy).

They may be more erratic, so that different variations of normal beats, followed by the disrhythmic beats are occurring.

Some people may experience several PVCs/PACs in a row (i.e. couplets = 2, triplets = 3, etc...) but even experiencing multiples is not of concern, unless a run of them remains sustained/constant for more than 30 seconds at a time, with no normal heartbeats in-between, which would then fall under the category of "tachycardia". In most cases, runs of skip heartbeat palpitations, fall under the category of "Non-Sustained Ventricular Tachycardia" (NSVT) and even this is usually considered a harmless event if the non-sustained periods are not frequent or occurring for more than 30 seconds at a time.

While statistics vary, some medical sources believe that half of us experience these sometimes irritating palpitations (likely closer to 100%) and that only about 30% actually notice them. Most doctors will not give them much credence, unless a patient also complains that the ectopic heartbeats are accompanied by significant lightheadedness, fainting, shortness of breath or chest pain.

If a patient complains about one of these co-morbid symptoms, a doctor might recommend cardiac testing or a visit to a heart specialist. In many cases, the symptoms are not directly related to the palpitations but may be a manifestation of co-occurring anxiety or from an unrelated health disorder (i.e. acid reflux, asthma or joint/muscle pain). Even without significant co-morbid symptoms, some patients will need to see a cardiologist, in order to experience peace-of-mind, knowing that they have good heart-health and that the palpitations will not lead to any serious event. The disrhythmias can be of slightly-higher concern when experienced by the elderly, by those with hypertensive conditions (high blood pressure) or by those who have known heart problems but they otherwise pose no dangers to those who experience them, who are relatively heart-healthy.

I recently received a comment from a lady who read one of my resources that contained information on the PVC/PAC subject and she complained about my not offering more substantial information regarding how to get rid of them. I responded to her comment with the reply that follows. ---

My Reply:

"I felt it might add perspective to mention that there has so far not been a treatment developed that rids sufferers of PVCs, of their heart-skip palpitations (some patients are referred for "ablations"- destruction of small area of heart tissue but most doctors feel this is too-risky for benign heart palpitations -- same is true of drugs that are specifically-designed to control abnormal heart beats).

Certainly some people with the condition have found relief from certain things such as supplementing with omega-3 essential oils (fish oil caplets) potassium or magnesium; to relieve or completely resolve their PVCs but others trying these very same supplements and see little or see no improvement.

With this being the case, every book or info source you find on the subject, will contain basically the same information regarding lifestyle changes to improve PVCs, such as stress-reduction, exercise, beta-blockers, anti-anxiety drugs and avoiding stimulants in the diet.

Giving heart-skip palpitation sufferers reassurance that PVCs will not harm someone with a structurally normal heart is in my opinion, possibly the most effective method in helping them to cope with them and in some cases, this actually helps them to overcome them completely (in many cases this requires the aid of a psychologist).

The reason being that fear of PVCs actually triggers them because they can be fueled and literally caused by adrenaline surges, such as those experienced by anxiety disorder sufferers.

I -in-fact believe a PVC Syndrome should be included in the list of known, major anxiety disorders. While I do give the same type info found via online sources on the PVC subject in my articles and books/eBooks, I concentrate a great deal of the information on helping PVCers not fear the symptoms of these devilish little heart palpitations.

When it comes to health conditions and diseases, I personally have yet to find a book/eBook with information that is not already found online.

I also believe with firm conviction that this can serve as frustration to those who order a new health title and find that it repeats basically the same information they have previously found online, especially those with difficulty coping or who have severe cases of a particular health problem.

At the same time, there are those who are new to a health condition or who prefer not to conduct lengthy online search to connect the major info-aspects of a health disorder all together for a better perspective on them. If one is lucky, they find free online sources that do cover all major aspects of a subject but this is not usually the case and successful online search requires putting-in exactly-correct combinations of search terms, otherwise certain sets of information remain obscure. Sometimes, even the most obvious search-terms do not yield the specific information they are seeking (I have experienced this problem myself on many occasions).

There simply is no "magic bullet" for curing PVCs and I for one would love to see one be developed.

I am a patient who suffers with these and at times mine can be very frequent and sometimes concerning. The reassurance that they do not cause heart damage in those with otherwise normal hearts, has been a major help in coping for me personally."

End of Reply

CHAPTER TWO

Heart-Skip Palpitations (PVCs) and Cardiomyopathy

(Heart Enlargement Risk with Premature Ventricular Contractions?)

As noted earlier, according to reputable heart doctors about half (50%) of the population experiences PVC – heart-skip palpitations. Some people have them far more frequently than others due to factors such as anxiety/stress and use of stimulants.

The cardiomyopathy scare that some people with frequent PVCs have after online search can be easily remedied by asking their doctors for a simple BNP blood test (B-Type Naturietic Peptide). This test detects both restrictive and constrictive cardiomyopathy, which always presents with degrees of heart enlargement and has 98% accuracy, according to The Harvard Medical School. Cardiomyopathy is also called Chronic Heart Failure and Congestive Heart Failure.

Even mild cases of it can be detected via the BNP blood test, which is also not expensive to have done. Of course an echocardiogram is an even more detailed test for looking at the heart but not everyone has health insurance or can afford to see a cardiologist to have one performed.

BNP Normal Values

The BNP levels they look for in people with mild heart failure is "100" and above in a range of 0 to 100. This would indicate mild cardiomyopathy. If the result comes in at 300 to 600, this indicates moderate heart failure and results at above 600, indicate severe heart failure. I would strongly suspect that the 2% loss of accuracy out of 98% involves those readings that are close to borderline because the higher readings are certain for heart enlargement.

BNP is actually a hormone released from the brain, in response to added pressure of any kind on the heart muscle and it will elevate even if there is stress on only one heart valve, such as the left ventricle or even if a person has chronic untreated, severe hypertension that has placed added stress and pressure on the heart.

If chronic PVCs have done this same thing (likely extremely rare, unless other heart disease is also present), the BNP will elevate.

My BNP Test Results

I had the BNP test ordered by my doctor, one year ago, after I developed adult asthma, that I felt certain was due to my chronic GERD (acid reflux), which I have had most of my life. With the fact however that heart enlargement can also cause breathing problems (cardiac asthma), I had the test ordered, plus a chest x-ray, which showed normal size heart. My BNP result came back at "4", which I was very happy with.

A few weeks ago, I had the BNP repeated after the onset of my most recent phase of PVCs and my result was very low again, at "16" -- still far below the "100" upper-normal cut-off value. This despite weeks of increase in my daily walking routine (doubled my distance) and the fact that the blood was drawn in the afternoon, rather than in the morning as the previous one was. BNP, like other hormones, will fluctuate several points within a 24 hour period and it also increases naturally with age.

I'm close to the half-century mark age-wise myself, so I'm very happy with my two low readings over the one-year period I had them done.

Heart Failure Risk in PVC Sufferers with otherwise Normal Hearts

For those who may have had a bit of cyberchondria rise up in their anxiety-sensitive hearts regarding heart failure, resulting from online search regarding PVCs, I wanted to add this bit of information for balance. Also keep in mind that literally 100s of online posts have been published by PVC sufferers, who have them very frequently, for decades and they still report having healthy heart check-ups.

Those who do develop heart disease following years of PVCs, could have a number of other factors involved (i.e. smoking, morbid obesity, severe untreated hypertension, heart defects or they are elderly etc...) and the PVCs may have had little or no involvement in the development of their cardiac diseases.

When heart disease is actually present, PVCs can be of some concern (some doctors state only slightly higher risks), as can many other things that are of far-less concern in people with otherwise health hearts.

The Real Scoop Regarding Congestive Heart Failure (Cardiomyopathy)

I will now add information regarding Congestive Heart Failure, for those readers who would like to know what this illness is really all-about and how it manifests.

Congestive Heart Failure (CHF) is more common in people ages 65 and older but can affect people at any age who have defects or damage to their heart muscles. In most patients, CHF has a chronic course but can be reversed in some cases. Even when it remains chronic (ongoing) treatments can be administered to treat symptoms and to improve quality of life for CHF patients. In some cases, fluid may build in a patient's lungs and/or their heart may become enlarged but there are treatments to relieve symptoms caused by complications of CHF.

Symptoms of CHF

The symptoms can vary among individuals, but the ones that are typically experienced may include the following:

* Shortness of breath

* Wheezing and coughing

* Edema in the ankles and/or abdomen (swelling)

* Fatigue

* Heart enlargement

* Exercise intolerance

* Failure in other organs of the body (i.e. the kidneys, liver and brain)

These symptoms occur due to a weakening of the heart muscle over time, which causes inadequate supply of blood circulation to the muscles and organs of the body. A resulting effect of diminished heart function out-put, includes a build-up of fluid around the heart and in the lungs, which also contributes to symptoms.

Causes of CHF

Conditions that cause serious heart arrhythmias (rather than the benign types) and damage to the heart muscle can result in the development of CHF over time. If a person has a severe heart murmur or a birth defect in the heart, for example (congenital heart defect) this can cause the condition to develop as they age and especially when they reach their senior-age years.

Heart attacks can also contribute to the development of CHF due to the resulting damage in the heart muscle that causes less-adequate heart function as a person ages. As the heart muscle struggles to supply proper blood circulation output while it is in a damaged or inadequately functioning state, it will often become enlarged. This is its attempt to allow more blood-flow through the heart valves but is a serious development that can require emergency care.

Lifestyle Treatments for CHF

If the condition is mild to moderate and not causing significant symptoms, a treating doctor might simply prescribe lifestyle changes.

Intermittent short-term use of a diuretic medication (for fluid retention) might also be recommended.

These changes in lifestyle might include the following:

* Losing excess weight in the body

* Regular exercise at proper tolerance level

* A healthy diet

* Reduced fluid intake

* Removing sodium from the diet (salt – which results in fluid retention)

This type of regimen would be monitored closely by regular follow ups with the patient, to see if the treatment is working or if prescription medications need to be added.

Prescription and Surgical Treatments

Prescribed medications for more severe cases of CHF, might include beta-blocker drugs to control hypertension and cardiac glycosides to increase cardiac output.

ACE Inhibitors might also be prescribed to prevent renin released by the kidneys from converting into angiotensin II (a hormone that causes heart constriction).

Should CHF worsen despite prescribed treatments, these worst-case scenarios might require corrective surgery for damaged or malfunctioning heart valves or for stints to be implanted to open constricted arteries. Rarely, a patient will be recommended for heart transplant if they are determined to be an approved candidate for one, meaning they are otherwise healthy, so that their body will not reject the replaced organ.

In many cases, the prognosis for CHF can be good with proper treatment and with close monitoring of treated patients by a qualified MD or cardiologist.

CHAPTER THREE

Do PVCs and PACs Increase the Risk for Premature Death?

(The Fear caused by Frequent Skips and Thumps)

I would hope to provide further comfort to those who experience these common heart palpitations, with frequency but I would also recommend that a medical doctor be consulted for further reassurance,when one is experiencing an irregular heartbeat of any type. While most heart palpitations are benign (harmless) some can indicate a structural problem within the heart muscle that requires treatment.

Skips and Thumps

PVCs and PACs are often felt by the one experiencing them, as a pause in the heartbeat, followed by a thump sensation in the chest, neck or abdomen and they are very common as previously mentioned. Due to the fact that they are experienced by such a large portion of the general population, huge numbers of posts regarding them can be found on heart-health medical forums online.

In some cases, patients are warning their fellow-patients, about the risk these palpitations have for causing eventual heart failure or sudden death from cardiac arrest. This type of information does however need to be seasoned with some perspective, based on reliable medical information, so as not to be ambiguous regarding realistic risk factors.

Many PVC/PAC Patients Report Good Heart Health

According to the information I found on reputable medical sources, regarding these common heart palpitations, heart disease **is not** the most common cause of PVCs/PACs. If that were the case, the estimated 50% of the general population, estimated to have relatively frequent PVCs/PACs, would all be walking around with heart disease. I have seen literally 1,000s of posts by frequent PVC/PAC sufferers, whose cardiologists ruled out structural heart disease of any kind via complete workups (i.e. stress test/EKG and echocardiograms) and yet they experience these horrible-feeling pause-thumps, on a daily bases.

Many relate having experienced them since their childhood and yet they were still given a clean bill of heart health in their 30s, 40s or 50s, by their cardiologists.

More on Palpitations and Cardiomyopathy

In regard to cardiomyopathy, which was discussed in a previous chapter (weakening of the heart muscle), PVCs/PACs should not place any more stress on the heart than would normal activities that increase the heart rate (i.e. exercise, excitement and sex), because the premature beat that happens with PVCs/PACs, is simply that...a double-beat. This would be equal to two heartbeats that simply occur closer together.

People who do develop cardiomyopathy with years of constant PVCs/PACs, likely had a propensity or predisposition toward developing it and the palpitations were simply a contributing factor. I will add that in rare cases, it's possibly a direct cause of heart failure but likely far more of a possibility in senior age people and/or in those who already have serious co-morbid health problems.

I base this on my search/research on many medical websites that specialize in heart health information. I recently viewed a YouTube video by Dr. Stephen Sinatra, a Board Certified Cardiologist, in which he states these facts, plus admits the he also experiences PVCs, as did many of his fellow students, which they discovered when they were studying for their medical credentials. He mentions "stress" in the video, as a precipitating factor for the occurrence of these palpitations, in students pursuing their educational degrees to practice professional medicine.

The Diagnostic Value of Common Irregular Heartbeats

Far too many reputable cardiologists are stating that their many years as practitioners in this field of specialty have shown that these irregular heartbeats are very common and very rarely pose a health threat to otherwise healthy people (some cardiologists even call them "normal"). They add statements to this fact, saying to the effect that PVCs/PACs rarely have any diagnostic significance and many of these doctors admit to experiencing them their selves.

Keep in mind that we are talking about irregular heartbeats, rather than chronic arrhythmias (an ongoing rather than intermittent change in cardiac rhythm).

Stress and Anxiety: Major Triggers for Palpitations

I also want to remind, that people, who anticipate PVCs/PACs, due to their fear of them, are actually contributing to more of them (certainly not their fault but a natural response).

Also, when one occurs, it tends to cause a quick surge of adrenaline in the body, due to the anxiety these palpitations may cause (fight or flight response) and this will instantly trigger succeeding PVCs/PACs, possibly several of them in a row.

For this reason, people who are under chronic stress or anxiety can experience them with more frequency than do people who have other triggers for them (i.e. caffeine, following exercise or lack of sleep).

Cardiologist - Dr. Michael G. Kienzle, MD says this regarding PVCs:

"...PVCs are common. In the vast majority of cases, they are of no prognostic significance and frequently go away on their own without any treatment beyond being reassured by your doctor."

While it is my hope that this chapter has also provided a bit of comfort to those who may be experiencing these skips and jumps in their heart rhythm, I do want to again remind that any type of heart arrhythmia should be further evaluated by a qualified doctor, as a wise precaution.

CHAPTER FOUR

Common Treatments for Heart Palpitations

(Lifestyle, Pharmaceutical and Natural Solutions for PVCs and PACS)

Magnesium and Potassium Supplementation

Studies of people with PVCs and PACs have revealed that they are often low in one or both of these essential minerals that have a great deal to do with healthy heart function. When these necessary elements in the body become low or are at sub-normal levels, this can contribute to arrhythmias such as tachycardia, skipped beats, flip-flops and flutters. Taking a safe supplementation-dose of magnesium and/or potassium as overseen by a medical professional, may help to control these symptoms and also contribute to overall better heart-health. To determine if a patient with palpitations is low in magnesium and/or potassium, a qualified doctor would first need to order mineral analysis tests, by blood or hair sample.

Beta-blocker Medications

Beta-adrenergic blocking agents or "beta-blockers" are medications that control blood pressure irregularities, especially hypertension (high blood pressure) which can also be a co-occurring symptom or even a cause of heart palpitations. It can also help to regulate blood pressure changes that patients with palpitations can experience with positional changes of their body or their "postural blood pressure". In addition to this, the medication can help reduce spells of tachycardia and diminish the effects of anxiety and panic symptoms that are experienced, by blocking some of the effects of adrenaline that tends to be overactive in many patients with skipped heartbeats and rapid heart rate.

Avoid Stimulants

Patients who experience concerning palpitations need to reduce or completely eliminate the amount of stimulants in their diets. These would be things including alcohol, caffeine, and refined sugar (added sugar not occurring naturally in foods).

Elimination of these can help control symptoms of anxiety and arrhythmias and help to keep stress-levels down which can also contribute to symptoms.

Reduce Stress and Drink Water

Stress, in fact is also a stimulant that needs to be reduced as much as possible due to its effect in also contributing-to and aggravating heart palpitations. Patients with bothersome palpitations should also remain well-hydrated, meaning they should drink plenty of water which helps to keep blood volume at the correct level. If there is not adequate water intake, blood volume can drop, causing a condition called "hypovolemia", which can contribute to symptoms of fatigue, dizziness and heart rhythm disturbances.

The Benefits of Regular Exercise

Regular exercise at a safe pace and at a well-tolerated level can also reduce stress and help to keep the involuntary nervous system better balanced in regulating blood pressure and heart rhythm.

Exercise has also been found in research studies to help reduce anxiety and depression levels, as well as-do medications that are also designed for this.

Should a patient with frequent PVCs or PACS also need the help of an anti-anxiety or antidepressant medication or emotional therapies these should also be considerations in helping them to cope with symptoms and to regain a better quality-of-life.

Types of anti-anxiety medications (benzodiazepines) include the following:

• alprazolam (Xanax®)

• clonazepam (Klonipin®)

• lorazepam (Ativan®)

• diazepam (Valium®)

• buspirone (Buspar®) (this one is a azaspirodecanedione class drug)

Types of anti-depressants (selective serotonin reuptake inhibitors) that also work as anti-anxiety medications include the following:

• paroxetine (Paxil®)

• venlafexine (Effexor®)

• fluoxetine (Prozac®)

• setraline (Zoloft®)

• fluvoxamine (Luvox ®)

In regard to psychiatric therapies, one that is highly successful in treating anxiety disorders and conditions of all kinds is "Cognitive Behavioral Therapy" (CBT). This method can be administered by a qualified mental health professional or in some cases; it can be self-administered via programs than can be used in the privacy of one's home. I do suggest however that home programs found by online search or at bookstores, have the endorsement or involvement of a psychiatric doctor or a reputable mental health association.

Get Complete Blood Tests

As previously mentioned, minerals such as magnesium and potassium can become low in the body. These are also in the "electrolyte" category and several other nutrients are as well, including phosphate and sodium.

Imbalances in these can affect heart function as well if they fall significantly outside of normal values -- whether levels become abnormally low or abnormally high in the body.

Blood tests can also detect abnormal levels of vitamins (i.e. B12, D and B6) and hormone levels (i.e. sex, adrenal and thyroid hormones), all of which can also affect heart function when they become significantly imbalanced.

Hyperthyroidism for example (overactive thyroid gland), can cause heart palpitations, such as sustained tachycardia and correction of the hormone imbalance can restore normal heart rhythm. These reasons are why it is important to ask one's doctor for complete blood tests, to detect potential causes of heart palpitations.

This will allow-for treatment of such underlying causes that might be found, which can improve or even completely correct the occurrence of PVCs, PACs and other common heart arrhythmias.

In Conclusion:

These often concerning but common and treatable heart palpitations do not have to disrupt a person's life any more than necessary, when methods for identifying causes or contributing factors are used, followed by administration of best-possible treatments for them. In many cases, self-administered lifestyle changes can greatly assist in treatment, in addition to that which may be required under the supervision of a medical doctor. In-short, sufferers of frequent PVCs and PACs can be assured that they will recover quality-of-life by being proactive in their treatment.

I offer my sincerest "Best Wishes" to the readers of this section, who undertake such remedies for their benign but emotionally-impacting heart palpitations and I thank you for reading the information I have offered!
(END - SECTION TWO)

SECTION THREE:

Cardiac Effects of Hypothyroidism and Hyperthyroidism

Heart Problems caused by Thyroid Disease

TABLE OF CONTENTS:

INTRODUCTION:

Thyroid disease is a major contributor to heart conditions of various types and can manifest as either hypothyroid or hyperthyroid disorders. This is why it is very important for both men and women (especially women), to be checked for abnormal thyroid hormone levels, beginning at age 35. A check for developing hypothyroidism or hyperthyroidism should also be done, at any point in life regardless of age, when symptoms of either condition appear to be developing.

Catching and treating thyroid disorders at their earliest stages, can help to prevent associated heart conditions from also developing or from worsening if already present. When people become thyroid hormone imbalanced, this can also exacerbate an already existing cardiac condition, which also means that treatments determined to be needed, by a qualified medical doctor or doctors (plural in cases when both an endocrinologist and cardiologist are needed), require more diligence on the part of both patient and physician, in order to extend life-expectancy and to maintain a better quality of life.

Within the chapters that follow, I will be addressing the types of heart conditions or cardiac effects that thyroid diseases can have on those who experience them. I will also discuss the treatments in-general, that are administered to correct or to help control these potentially serious problems. It is my sincere hope that this resource helps to provide a worthy general educational resource for its readers.

-*Jim Lowrance*

CHAPTER ONE

Hypercholesterolemia from Underactive Thyroid Gland

Hypothyroidism is the second leading cause of high cholesterol (Hypercholesterolemia), second-only to bad diet practices. This fatty substance that is found in the body, is actually a necessary type of fat molecule, that keeps tissues healthy throughout the body, when present at the proper levels (i.e. not too high and not too low, depending on the type being referenced).

Cholesterol Aids in the Manufacture of Steroid Hormones

This essential fat molecule is also the substance that helps convert adrenal hormones into other needed steroid hormones (sterones), including those that moderate sexual identity and functions. Without the needed manufactured hormones that result from conversion of them, via cholesterol, there would also be a problem with sodium and water balance in the body, the immune system could not operate properly and inflammation could not be moderated in the body without the aid of this essential precursor element.

Without its help, stress hormones (the major one being "cortical") would also not be present to keep the body from succumbing to chronic or traumatic stressors and experiencing even mild stress would become intolerable both mentally and physically.

Conversion of Sunlight into Vitamin D

Another steroid hormone of great importance, that could not be manufactured for use in the body without cholesterol, is "vitamin D", which was only recently recognized for its steroid effect, in addition to its value as a vitamin. Cholesterol is the substance that converts sunlight into vitamin D in the body as well, to be used for keeping bones, muscles and nerves healthy. Of course we also receive the nutrient from foods we consume but medical research has recently found that both proper diet and ample sunlight may not even be enough to boost proper levels of the nutrient within the body and so supplementation with the vitamin may also be necessary for many individuals. Without the aid of cholesterol however, vitamin D would have to be mega-supplemented as a lifelong practice.

High Cholesterol and Atherosclerosis

While the previously described positive effects, result from proper good cholesterol levels in the body, when the bad type becomes abnormally elevated, it can begin to stick to the walls of the arteries, throughout the body, as a type of "plaque". This is a condition referred to as "atherosclerosis" and the resulting effect of this condition includes a narrowing of blood flow through affected arteries and a hardening of them. If arteries leading to the heart become severely narrowed or completely blocked, this can result in a heart attack or heart failure and most-often in hypertension (high blood pressure) in its early stages.

If the arteries leading from the heart to other parts of the body become affected, this can cause tissues starved of proper blood-nourishment, to become inoperable (paralyzed), including the arms or legs, which can be the result of a condition referred to as "Peripheral Artery Disease" (PAD), often beginning as a painful malady, that can also result in dangerous blood-clotting.

When atherosclerosis from hypercholesterolemia results in loss of blood supply to the brain, due to major arteries supplying blood to the organ being blocked, a stroke can be the result. In worse case scenarios, heart attacks and strokes can be fatal or can leave the afflicted person in a brain-vegetated state. Even in milder cases, a person can be left with varied degrees of brain damage and/or heart damage/failure.

Lipid Screenings and Thyroid Panels

These facts demonstrate the importance in regular lipid screenings (blood tests), to check for imbalances of either too-high a level of the cholesterol that can become bad for the body ("LDL" - low density lipoproteins) and/or too-low a level of the type that is good for the body ("HDL" - high density lipoproteins). This becomes more important when men and women reach ages 35 and older. If hypercholesterolemia is diagnosed (high LDL), it also becomes important to find the cause of the condition, so that it can be corrected to the fullest-extent (i.e. determining if there are contributing disorders, such as thyroid disease needing treatment).

In many cases an underlying cause may seem obvious, such as apparent morbid obesity however, weight gain can be the result of hypothyroidism, as well as the cause of high cholesterol. With this being the case, blood testing of thyroid hormone levels should also be ordered, rather than taking-for-granted that <u>the cause</u> of imbalanced lipid levels is already apparent. A grouping of blood tests called a "thyroid panel" can be ordered with the simple stroke-of-a-pen by a doctor, to rule-out or to confirm thyroid involvement.

While some patients in-whom a thyroid disease is missed due to a lack of testing, can actually see improvement in their hypercholesterolemia by being prescribed a medication for the condition called a "statin drug" (HMG-CoA reductase inhibitor), this <u>would not</u> correct the underlying hypothyroidism or the other harmful effects that can result from it over time. Treatment specifically for the underactive thyroid would also be necessary, to prevent further serious health consequences.

Hypothyroidism an Elusive cause of Hypercholesterolemia (Medical Research)

Following is a quote from medical research published on the PubMed website (U.S. National Institutes of Health), regarding hypothyroidism not always being an apparent/obvious cause ofhyperchortisolemia:

"Hypothyroidism is a cause of secondary hyperlipidaemia. This study investigates the frequency of biochemically diagnosed hypothyroidism and its relationship with plasma cholesterol concentration in apparently healthy people.

Thyroid function tests (total T4, TSH, and free T4) were performed on 272 apparently healthy men and women (179 vegetarians, 93 meat eaters) with a plasma cholesterol concentration above 7 mmol/l and on 90 individuals with a plasma cholesterol below 4.1 mmol/l who were matched for age, sex and dietary habits.

Six per cent of those with a plasma cholesterol above 7 mmol/l had biochemical evidence of hypothyroidism as defined by a TSH greater than 10 mIU/l (reference range 1-6) ---

---

and a low free T4 below 10pmol/l (reference range 10.1-25). Eighty per cent of these people had a high titre of thyroid anti-microsomal antibodies. Of the 90 individuals with a plasma cholesterol level below 4.1 and the 25 randomly selected participants none had biochemical evidence of hypothyroidism.

Hypothyroidism is relatively common in apparently healthy people with a raised plasma cholesterol. It appears no commoner in vegetarians than in meat eaters."

(From the Article Titled: **"Asymptomatic hypothyroidism and hypercholesterolaemia."** - Online Link Location: http://www.ncbi.nlm.nih.gov/pmc/articles/PMC12 93411/

Treating High Cholesterol in Hypothyroid Patients

In many cases of only mild to moderately elevated cholesterol in a newly diagnosed hypothyroid patient, treatment by their doctor, with thyroid hormone replacement therapy will resolve the issue.

His will occur once the hormones reach adequate and preferably "optimal levels" (suppressing TSH and raising T4 and T3 levels into the higher range of normal). NOTE: "TSH" is a pituitary hormone that <u>elevates</u> with hypothyroidism, while the "T4 and T3" levels are the actual thyroid hormones that do the opposite of TSH and drop <u>below normal</u> with an underactive thyroid. The goal of hypothyroid treatment is to return each of these back to best-possible normal ranges.

If however, the cholesterol elevation is severe and/or a patient is also significantly obese or suffers from another endocrine disorder such as diabetes, other treatments may also be required, such as a prescribed statin drug as mentioned previously. Lifestyle changes would also likely be recommended by a treating doctor as well, even with normalized cholesterol levels, such as avoidance of a high-fat diet or one that indulges in the consumption of too much refined sugar (the manufactured types, that can highly increase triglycerides) and an increase in healthy foods that contain high-fiber content (i.e. fruits, vegetables, nuts and grains).

An increase in physical activity, such as a well-tolerated aerobic exercises would likely also be recommended (i.e. walking, jogging or bicycling). Encouraging patients to practice stress-reduction methods might also be an added feature of treatment, due to the opinion by some medical experts, that high stress levels can actually contribute to increased bad cholesterol in the body.

Highly activated stress hormones, can cause low reserves of them over time, leaving the body vulnerable to inflammation and an increase in fat storage by the body as it senses a chronic stress emergency (some sources refer to this as "adrenal fatigue").

Patients who smoke might be referred to programs to help them quit, since smoking can directly, negatively affect cholesterol metabolism in the body.

If the good "HDL" cholesterol level in a patient has dropped below normal, a doctor might also recommend that they take a daily fish oil supplement (a source of omega-3 fatty acids), which acts like the mechanism of good cholesterol, by helping to clear any excess LDL level from the arteries, thereby returning it to the liver, to be flushed as waste from the body. While cholesterol is essential to the body, it is important to keep both the good and bad levels of it, as well-balanced as possible for a healthier life.

CHAPTER TWO

Thyrotoxicity and Heart Arrhythmias

To become "thyrotoxic", can mean a number of things but a general understanding of the term would be "hyperthyroidism" (excessive thyroid hormone).

Causes of Thyrotoxicity

In most cases of thyrotoxicity, the cause is a disease process within the thyroid gland, such as the autoimmune condition called "Graves' disease" (over 90% of cases) or the development of tumors within the gland called "thyroid nodules" and more specifically those referred to as "hot nodules", which manufacture thyroid hormone just as natural thyroid tissue does but at abnormally high amounts. People can become overcharged with thyroid hormones for other reasons as well, including that which results from taking doses of thyroid hormone replacement (therapy for hypothyroidism), at excessively high amounts or due to over-supplementing with iodine that is an ingredient in a medication or in a natural supplement.

This can also include the consumption of large amounts of high-iodine content foods such as kelp (a type of seaweed - 1 tablespoon contains about 2000/mcg of iodine).

Manifestations of Being Thyrotoxic

The resulting effect of hyperthyroidism, is a bodily metabolism that is sped up to an abnormally high level. This will cause the person experiencing it, to feel high energy levels because the body will burn fuel coming into it (foods consumed), at an excessive rate. When this occurs, the following symptoms may result as shown below (some people will experience only some of these, depending on how severe the hyperthyroidism/thyrotoxicity is).

• Very high energy levels

• Diarrhea

• Anxiety and nervousness

• Increased Sweating

• Insomnia

• Hyperventilation (over-breathing)

• Hypertension (high blood pressure)

• Tachycardia episodes (spells of rapid heart rate)

• Muscle wasting

• Lack of nutrient retention (from chronic diarrhea)

• Bone loss (osteoporosis)

Two of the symptoms listed above (hypertension and tachycardia episodes), are the ones that have an effect on heart rhythm. Hypertension is a known cause for triggering abnormal heart beats over time but even apart from the high blood pressure, the person experiencing a hyperthyroid condition will experience episodes of tachycardia. When these two symptoms are combined, this increases the chances for the tachycardia to evolve into more serious types of chronic (sustained) heart arrhythmias.

These would include "Super Ventricular Tachycardia" (SVT), which originates from the lower chambers of the heart and "Paroxysmal Atrial Tachycardia" (PAT), which originates from the upper chambers of the heart.

If treatment to control or to resolve the thyrotoxicity is not administered and is allowed to continue, potentially fatal heart arrhythmias can eventually occur (rare), such as "Atrial Fibrillation" (more common and not usually life threatening) or "Ventricular Fibrillation" (episodes can cause fainting or sudden, fatal cardiac arrest). As SVT and/or PAT occur, a person may experience the symptoms listed, following.

• Angina (chest pain)

• Palpitations (strong sensations of heart beat)

• Dizziness

• Shortness of breath

• Sweating

• Syncope (fainting or near fainting)

Treatments for Thyrotoxicity

In order to control or to resolve heart arrhythmias caused by thyrotoxic conditions, the excessive levels of thyroid hormone in the body will need to be lowered back down into the normal range to restore a proper level of bodily metabolism. If excessive iodine or oral thyroid hormone is the culprit, simply reducing or eliminating these, can resolve the heart palpitations and arrhythmias that are occurring.

If a prescribed medication is involved, this will require the supervision of a medical doctor who can adjust a patient's dose, prescribe an alternative drug or add a new prescription to control this side effect, when a prescribed medication is mandatory and not able to be changed or stopped.

When hyperthyroidism caused by a condition such as Graves' disease is present, a doctor may prescribe one of a number of different anti-thyroid drugs ("thionamides" - those that lower thyroid hormone production).

This would include drugs such as Methimazole (MMI) and Propylthiouracil (PTU). Another drug that may be prescribed, to control hypertension and tachycardia is a "beta-blocker", which reduces the effects of adrenaline on the cardiovascular system and may include brands such as Atenolol or Metoprolol. Some hyperthyroid patients require a combination of both a beta-blocker and an anti-thyroid drug.

When a doctor determines that a diseased thyroid gland will not be controlled well-enough through medication treatment alone, he may refer a patient to a thyroid surgeon for removal of their gland (total thyroidectomy) or partial removal of their gland (sub-total thyroidectomy).

A partial removal is usually the case when only one lobe of the gland is affected by a hot nodule, while total removal is often the case with Graves' disease patients (another term for the disease is "toxic diffuse goiter" - meaning the entire gland is affected).

Another option however, is for the patient's gland to be "ablated", meaning it is destroyed via radioactive iodine, that is administered to the patient at a high-enough dose to fully eradicate all thyroid tissue from the body ("RAI" - Radioactive Iodine Ablation).

Treatment also becomes a priority due to tachycardia and other heart arrhythmias posing a risk for the development of an enlarged heart (Chronic Heart Failure) and/or a heart attack. In many cases, resolving the thyrotoxicity gives the heart opportunity to partially or fully recover from any enlargement or damage it has experienced.

Following is a PubMed medical research article quote, stating that atrial fibrillation is the most common type of heart arrhythmia associated with throtoxicity:

BACKGROUND:

Cardiac arrhythmias associated with thyrotoxicosis tend to be supraventricular in nature with atrial fibrillation being the most common.

Ventricular arrhythmias are rarely associated with thyrotoxicosis and are considered to be secondary to intrinsic cardiac disease.

SUMMARY:

We present three patients with thyrotoxicosis and stable coronary disease in whom the primary cardiac rhythm disturbance was ventricular tachycardia. In all of these patients, the ventricular arrhythmias terminated with achievement of a euthyroid state. We hypothesize that the thyrotoxic state contributed to the etiology of, or lowered the threshold for the ventricular arrhythmias.

CONCLUSION:

Prompt attention to the management of thyrotoxicosis in patients with a history of significant heart disease is warranted in order to avoid potentially fatal arrhythmias.

(From the Article Titled: **"Thyrotoxicosis-induced ventricular arrhythmias."** - Link: http://www.ncbi.nlm.nih.gov/pubmed/18816176)

Keep in mind when considering the facts stated in the above-quoted medical research, that tachycardia (rapid heartbeat) is very common with hyperthyroid conditions but it is not always considered an arrhythmia in the same sense as those described within the article. Tachycardia is also very common in other conditions such as anxiety disorders however, chronic anxiety or panic attacks do not cause a sustained type of severe tachycardia and seldom lead to actual heart conditions.

A resting heart rate above 100 beats per minute is determined to be higher-than-normal, whether sustained or intermittent. This type of problem is often called a "palpitation" however, severe tachycardia that is prolonged (chronic), such as that occurring with untreated thyrotoxic states, can eventually lead to cardiomyopathy (heart failure) and enlargement of the heart as the valves within it, begin to stretch excessively due to the added strain placed upon them (valvular heart disease).This is why treating hyperthyroidism as early as possible, becomes important.

CHAPTER THREE

Hyperthyroid and Hypothyroid Cardiomyopathy

Within the previous chapters, reference was made to "cardiomyopathy" and "heart enlargement" however, while these conditions are often directly associated with each other, they are actually two different things.

What is Cardiomyopathy?

Cardiomyopathy actually is a term simply meaning that the heart muscle has become weakened for whatever reason, whether it be due to a disease process, chronic lack of oxygen or extremely strenuous activity placed upon the heart muscle.

If for example, in a disease process, there is a connective-tissue disorder occurring within the body, such as Systemic Lupus Erythematosus ("SLE"- a body wide autoimmune condition), the heart can eventually become affected, leading to a weakening of the organ (this can also be true in some cases of Rheumatoid Arthritis and Sjögren's Syndrome).

If the scenario of prolonged hypoxia has occurred, meaning lack of oxygen in the body, such as that which occurs in people suffering from pulmonary (lung) disorders, this can eventually lead tocardiomyopathy as well (i.e. types of COPD, Lung Fibrosis and Lung Cancer).

If yet another scenario occurs, such as athletes who extend, excessively-added strain on the heart (beyond healthy levels) their hearts can eventually become weakened, rather than strengthened because they have gone beyond the muscle's tolerance level for extended periods of time. This has been reported to happen to pro football and basketball players, and to pro wrestlers, who have over-trained their bodies for many years, to reach peak performance and appearance levels however, their hearts were not given time to rest and repair and so they eventually became weakened as a result. This has also been found to be the case in athletes who have taken anabolic steroids to increase muscle size and strength, which placed undue strain on the heart muscle, leading to eventual cardiomyopathy.

The symptoms of cardiomyopathy may include the following:

- Fatigue and easy fatigability

- Shortness of breath

- Chest pain or discomfort

- Cardiac arrhythmias and/or palpitations

What is Heart Enlargement?

In the case of heart enlargement (also covered in a previous section/chapter), the muscle expands to sizes that are outside of normal values, which can be due to a number of reasons as well. A major cause of heart enlargement however, is cardiomyopathy because when the heart weakens, it has to work harder to perform the same task of supplying blood-flow to every part of the body.

Other causes or contributing-factors for heart enlargement, also referred to as "Chronic Heart Failure" (CHF), can include the following, as listed on the nest page. ---

---

• Diseases affecting heart valves (including severe Mitral Valve Prolapse)

• Severe untreated hypertension

• Heart damage (i.e. heart attack)

• Chronic Anemia

• Iron excess (hemochromatosis)

• Congenital heart defects (problems at birth)

• Morbid obesity

• Cigarette smoking

• Metabolic diseases (i.e. thyroid and diabetic disorders)

As this struggle with the heart continues, the heart attempts to compensate by widening its valves, which causes them to stretch. If this stretching of the heart is caught early enough, it can actually be reversed in some cases however, like a rubber band that only has so much elasticity, the valves and muscle can become stretched to the point that the enlargement cannot be reversed or can only be partially reversed.

At this point, a treating doctor will attempt to halt further enlargement from occurring or to at least slow it down as much as possible.

When the heart enlarges, the same symptoms can occur that were listed previously for cardiomyopathy however, as the enlargement progresses, other symptoms, such as fluid retention in parts of the body ("edema" - swelling) will occur, most-often beginning in the feet and lower-legs but that can also manifest in the mid-section of the body and in the hands.

Patients with CHF may also develop breathing difficulties, such as asthmatic symptoms (cardiac asthma) and difficulty breathing after becoming supine for several minutes or hours ("orthopnea" - shortness of breath when laying flat).

They may also hear noticeable wheezing or bubbling sounds coming from their lungs at times, which is caused by pulmonary edema (lung fluid) that builds within breathing passages.

Diagnosis and Treatments for Cadiomyopathy and Heart Enlargement

A doctor may suspect that his patient has myopathy or enlargement of their heart, if any of the symptoms listed previously are occurring. The patient would then be referred for cardiac testing, such as an "electrocardiogram" ("EKG" - possibly the "stress test" version, with observation during exertion) and an "echocardiogram" (cardiac sonogram), which is a detailed sound-wave imaging of the heart, observed on a screen to observe its functioning.

In many cases, a typical chest x-ray (radiograph still image), will show any enlargement affecting certain valve areas or of the heart in general.

A particular blood test that has been recently recognized as being <u>very accurate</u> for detecting even mild heart enlargement, is one called the "B-type Natriuretic Peptide" ("BNP" - a hormone released from lower chambers of the heart if it experiences abnormal pressures).

The test, according to some medical sources, is up to 98% accurate in detecting CHF and the upper-normal, cut-off value is "<**100 pg/ml**", meaning any results of the blood test that yield a result at 100 and above, are strongly indicative of heart failure/enlargement. Some abnormal values charts published by medical sources, state that readings between 100 and 300 indicate mild CHF, readings between 300 and 600 indicate moderate cases, while those that are above 600, indicate severe heart failure (some patients see readings in the 1,000s).

The main focus when cardiomyopathy and/or heart enlargement is found, is to determine any underlying causes in order to treat them for control or elimination of them. This of course would include correcting thyrotoxic/hyperthyroid states, which will lift the excessive pressure from the heart, allowing it a degree of rest and repair (possible complete reversal). In addition to eliminating contributing factors to also include cessation of smoking and weight loss for obese patients, other things added to a treatment regimen by a patient's doctor, may include the following, as listed on the next page. ---

---

• Regular exercise at proper tolerance level

• A healthy diet

• Reduced fluid intake

• Removing sodium from the diet (salt – which results in fluid retention)

• Hypertensive medications

Following is a PubMed medical research article, that refers to "idiopathic dilated cardiomyopathy", as related to thyroid disorders.

"Severe thyrotoxicosis can cause irreversible congestive heart failure. To investigate the coincidence of subclinical thyroid disorders and idiopathic dilated cardiomyopathy (IDC) we investigated these patients with respect to their morphological and functional thyroid status. Thyroid sonography as well as thyroid hormone levels were measured in all patients.

RESULTS: Sixty-one patients (50 male, 11 female) with chronic stable IDC were included. Two out of 61 patients showed completely normal thyroid morphology and function. The other 59 patients showed either morphological or functional abnormalities or both. Of the 53 patients with morphological abnormalities 23 patients (all male) showed diffuse goiter as opposed to 29 nodular enlarged organs (24 male, 5 female). No clinically significant hypothyroidism or thyrotoxicosis was seen. A good correlation was found between the duration of IDC and thyroid volume (r = 0.44; p < 0.001). Two patients died during the study period, 1 from sudden death and 1 from progressive heart failure.

CONCLUSION: Subclinical thyroid disorders are frequently seen in patients with long-standing IDC when they live in an area of chronic iodine deficiency. This can be explained by chronic salt restriction as basic treatment for congestive heart failure. ...

...

Therefore we conclude that examination of the thyroid gland should be done routinely in patients with IDC, especially when restriction of salt intake is recommended by the treating physician."

(From the Article Titled: **"Subclinical thyroid disorders in patients with dilated cardiomyopathy."** - Online Link Location: http://www.ncbi.nlm.nih.gov/pubmed/9096916)

The preceding information clearly conveys the importance in getting thyrotoxic states normalized to prevent these types of cardiac issues from occurring or worsening.

CHAPTER FOUR

PVCs and PACs from Thyroid Hormone Imbalance

Premature Ventricular Contractions (PVCs) and Premature Atrial Contractions (PACs) are also referred to as "ectopic heartbeats".

What are PVCs and PACs and Why do They Occur?

These common and usually benign heart arrhythmias (also referred to as "dysrhythmias") are extra beats that are triggered by cells within the heart-muscle, located close to the lower chambers of the heart (the ventricles) or close to the upper chambers (the atria), that become excitable/charged with the ability to emit mild electrical impulses.

The heart normally beats as a result of its own electrical pacemaker system but the extra electrical impulses that occur with PVCs and PACs, actually add extra beats in-between those the natural pacemaker is already triggering.

Symptoms of Ectopic Heartbeats

In spite of these being <u>extra beats,</u> they will feel more like pauses in the heartbeat to the person who experiences them. After the pause-sensation, some people who experience ectopic heartbeats, also describe the feeling of an extra-hard beat following it, or what they might call a strong thump inside their chest. This is due to the very slightly added extra-time of only a second or two for the heart to fill-up with blood, so that when it fully contracts, there is slightly more blood being pushed-out. These sensations, that can also include feelings such as the heart fluttering, flip-flopping, pounding or slightly changing speeds, also places them in the "palpitations" category.

Some people with ectopic beats may report these other symptoms occurring with them as well:

• Anxiety or panic feelings

• Mild adrenaline surges

• Slight dizziness

• Minor chest pain or discomfort ...

...

- Head rush (sudden blush)

- Urge to cough

- Shortness of breath

- Mild headaches

- Insomnia

While PVCs and PACs are harmless in the vast majority of cases, some can be associated with serious heart conditions and should be evaluated by a medical doctor, as a precaution. This is especially true, if any of the symptoms listed-above become significant or if a patient has a past history of significant heart problems.

Most patients can be given the clear by their doctor, with a simple physical evaluation but if there is any suspicion for structural heart damage or abnormalities, a patient might be referred to a cardiologist or for diagnostic testing such as an EKG or echocardiogram.

Common Murmurs, Arrhythmias and Myopathies of the Heart

Some patients presenting with a variety of different palpitations, are discovered to have a common "click heart murmur" called "Mitral Valve Prolapse" ("MVP" - briefly referenced earlier in a list of possible causes for heart enlargement). The condition is common in the general population and slightly more common in thyroid patients but in the vast majority of cases it is benign and requires only lifestyle changes or a beta-blocker drug to help control any symptoms it is causing.

In severe cases of MVP, in which significant "mitral regurgitation" is present, surgery may be required to repair the faulty heart valve (rare). Otherwise, MVP-Syndrome (the "syndrome" suffix added when symptoms are present), is simply a condition that can be an annoyance to some patients but is rarely ever life-threatening and very seldom requires surgical intervention. The condition can however, cause or contribute to the frequency of PVCs and/or PACs in people who experience it.

Ectopic Beats Caused by Thyroid Hormone Imbalance

Among the causes of PVCs and PACS, are included things such as stress and anxiety, lack of sleep, intake of stimulants (i.e. tobacco, alcohol, caffeine and refined-sugar excess), increased exercise (during or following) and hormonal imbalances. Women report that ectopic beats can correlate with their menstrual cycles and pregnancies, and certainly with added stressors of any kind, the body can be flooded with more adrenal hormones (catecholamines). Another cause however, that has been reported by those who experience these palpitations that can be very annoying and sometimes very concerning to those who experience them, is "thyroid hormone imbalance".

While it is understandable that hyperthyroid patients would experience these dysrhythmias, with the added adrenaline in their bodies resulting from thyrotoxicity, patients with hypothyroidism also report experiencing them.

It's very possible that either abnormally low or abnormally high levels of hormones that are of any endocrine type (i.e. thyroid, adrenal, glucose regulating and the sex types), can potentially cause episodes of these added heartbeats. This can be true of natural hormones within the body that fluctuate and true of supplemented hormones, coming into the body from an outside source, if fluctuations in them occur as well.

Avoiding the Added Heartbeats as a Thyroid Patient

With hormones apparently playing a factor in these sometimes scary palpitations, one should not only avoid the triggers listed previously, such as added stressors, sleep deprivation and consuming too many stimulants (i.e. caffeinated coffee/tea, alcoholic beverages and manufactured sugars), one should also attempt to keep their hormones properly balanced as best possible. This would include thyroid hormones that are being taken as replacement therapy for hypothyroidism.

In order to accomplish this, hypothyroid patients should report any symptom-changes in their treated underactive thyroid conditions, to their doctors, in case a new blood test needs ordered sooner than scheduled to determine if a dose-change in the therapy is needed.

The daily dose prescribed should be taken faithfully,usually first thing in the morning on an empty stomach (at least 30 minutes before eating), with plenty of water to help it absorb into the system. Any supplements or foods with high calcium or any iron in them, should not be consumed until 6 hours after a thyroid dose is ingested (these can hinder its absorption).

While some patients develop hypothyroidism as the direct result of a disease within their glands, others develop it as the expected after-effect of treatments for hyperthyroidism (i.e. following thyroidectomies or RAI ablations). Either way, thyroid hormone replacement therapy is the required life-long treatment, for which there is no alternative.

Patients whose hypothyroid therapies are well-regulated as reflected by optimal normal-values blood test results of their TSH, T3 and T4 levels, only need retested, every 4 to 6 months once a euthyroid state is achieved (normalized metabolism). Testing may need to be repeated sooner however, if symptoms manifest between blood retests that are scheduled this far ahead and this should include the onset of heart palpitations of any type.

Not only can ectopic heartbeats signal an abnormal change in thyroid hormone levels but other types of palpitations can as well, including tachycardia (possibly indicating over-treatment with thyroid hormone) and "bradycardia" (a slowed heart rate, possibly indicating under-treatment). NOTE: Bradycardia is defined as a resting heart rate of below 60 beats per minute.

If additional medical treatment is needed for heart palpitations, this will usually be a beta-blocker medication and lifestyle changes, as discussed within the previous chapters.

There are different classes of "anti-arrhythmic drugs" available however, doctors usually prescribe these for the more serious types of heart arrhythmias rather than for ectopic beats which are usually not considered a risk-factor for anything potentially serious in otherwise heart-healthy individuals.

Some patients with serious types of arrhythmias are also referred to an electrophysiologist, which is a cardiologist who specializes in the electrical system of the heart. The specialist might then opt to perform what is referred-to as a "Radio frequency ablation" (RFA). This is a procedure in which a catheter, is inserted into the area of the heart where an arrhythmia originates-from and an electrode contained inside the catheter, transmits radio waves that ablate (destroy) a small area of heart tissue.

This can stop the abnormal impulses being transmitted by the heart's natural pacemaker however, the procedure carries some risks and is very rarely recommended for people with benign PVCs and/or PACs.

Following is an interesting medical research study in regard to ectopic heartbeats associated with thyroid hormone replacement therapy (the thyroid hormone dose did not increase PVCs but did slightly increase PACs in some of the participants studied):

"Whether thyroid replacement therapy can trigger cardiac arrhythmias in patients with hypothyroidism is not known. In this prospective study, 24 h ambulatory electrocardiographic (ECG) monitoring was used to assess the frequency of atrial and ventricular premature beats in 25 patients with hypothyroidism (5 men and 20 women, aged 56 +/- 3 years) before and 3.5 +/- 0.5 months (mean +/- SEM) after thyroid replacement therapy. Plasma thyroid-stimulating hormone was 73.6 +/- 12.3 and 3.1 +/- 0.6 microU/ml and free thyroxine index was 2.4 +/- 0.4 and 9.8 +/- 0.9 micrograms/100 ml at baseline and after thyroid replacement therapy, respectively.

The frequency of ventricular premature beats was not affected by thyroid replacement therapy (from 273 +/- 221 at baseline to 352 +/- 235 beats/24 h after therapy), even in patients with frequent baseline arrhythmias.

In contrast, the frequency of atrial premature beats was slightly increased after thyroid replacement therapy (from 47 +/- 17 to 279 +/- 197 beats/24 h), largely as a result of changes seen in three patients. No patient developed new onset of sustained ventricular or supraventricular arrhythmias.

Average, basal and maximal heart rates during ECG monitoring increased significantly after thyroid replacement therapy (average 72 +/- 2 to 80 +/- 2; basal 64 +/- 2 to 70 +/- 2; maximal 114 +/- 3 to 130 +/- 3 beats/min, respectively, p less than 0.001).

In conclusion, thyroid replacement therapy is safe in patients with common benign cardiac arrhythmias, and does not trigger an increase in arrhythmia frequency except in rare patients with baseline atrial premature beats.

It is, however, associated with an increase in basal, average and maximal heart rates."

(From the Article Titled: **"Effect of thyroid replacement therapy on the frequency of benign atrial and ventricular arrhythmias"** - Online Link Location: http://www.ncbi.nlm.nih.gov/pubmed/2477427)

Conclusion:

It is my hope that the information contained within this chapter and those within the sections that preceded it, have provided helpful information to readers seeking a general education regarding the more common cardiac manifestations that exist, in the form of murmurs, arrhythmias/dysrhythmias and myopathies.

(END)

ABOUT THE AUTHOR:

I am a husband, father, grandfather and lifetime contract salesman, with experience in health writing that began in 2004. I completed theological studies with Liberty University in 1996. I formerly served aseditor and forum moderator of Thyroid Health for a major multi-topic content site and as a general health writer for another, where I received Editor's Choice Awards for my articles on health subjects.

In 2003 I was diagnosed with hypothyroidism; "Hashimoto's thyroiditis" being the cause. This autoimmune form of thyroid disease that causes destruction of the thyroid gland resulted in my also developing "Chronic Fatigue Syndrome", due to a compromised immune system with severe co-morbid "Adrenal Fatigue". I also suffered severe anxiety symptoms, including panic attacks early into the onset of Hashimoto's thyroiditis (Hashitoxicosis). A common heart murmur I was diagnosed with in my teens called "Mitral Valve Prolapse", also worsened in severity of symptoms, with the development of these other health disorders.

My eventual receiving of diagnoses was a difficult process with proper diagnostic testing not being ordered by the first doctors I sought treatment from. These types of issues were inspiration for me to become proactive in my own health care and to self-educate myself on these health disorders, which I have done extensively since 2003. I now enjoy sharing this information with other patients experiencing my same health disorders.

During the early 1990s, I marketed an outdoors product I invented and that I formed a small corporation to patent, manufacture and sell called the "Rod Floater" (now a registered Trademark). I traveled the U.S. making presentations to groups of Wal-Mart zone and district managers and received authorization to sell the product in two regions of Wal-Mart stores for five years.

I also sold the product to Bass Pro Shops, Cabela's and Academy Stores, all of which still carry the product and I landed a national promotion for the product with Kerr-McGee Oil Company who began using the product to promote their outboard motor oil in 1992.

In 1996 I licensed the product to TTI-Blakemore, a major fishing tackle conglomerate, from which I am still paid royalties from sales of the product.

I invented and marketed five additional outdoors products, also getting these into Wal-Mart stores and afterward sold them outright rather than licensing them.

I was featured in the May 2001 issue of Inventors digest magazine.